Nesrine Kammoun
Wafa Elleuch

Educational sequence

Nesrine Kammoun
Wafa Elleuch

Educational sequence

Management of low back pain in working adults

ScienciaScripts

Imprint

Any brand names and product names mentioned in this book are subject to trademark, brand or patent protection and are trademarks or registered trademarks of their respective holders. The use of brand names, product names, common names, trade names, product descriptions etc. even without a particular marking in this work is in no way to be construed to mean that such names may be regarded as unrestricted in respect of trademark and brand protection legislation and could thus be used by anyone.

Cover image: www.ingimage.com

This book is a translation from the original published under ISBN 978-620-6-72186-4.

Publisher:
Sciencia Scripts
is a trademark of
Dodo Books Indian Ocean Ltd. and OmniScriptum S.R.L publishing group

120 High Road, East Finchley, London, N2 9ED, United Kingdom
Str. Armeneasca 28/1, office 1, Chisinau MD-2012, Republic of Moldova, Europe
Printed at: see last page
ISBN: 978-620-8-18616-6

Table of contents

INTRODUCTION

Medical training is a special kind of training, since it is particularly long, delivered by professionals and carried out both within the faculty and at the patient's bedside. The current teaching system, based largely on lectures, is often seen as boring, passive and inadequate, particularly when it comes to preparing for the specialist examination. The reform of the third cycle and the preparatory texts for its implementation emphasize the need to take into account the specific needs of each student, his or her career plans and any shortcomings in the training received previously (1).

Training can be based on either a skills-based or an objective-based approach.

The approach used in our teaching scenario is that of objectives. A learning objective is a statement that briefly describes what the student should be able to do after a learning process that he or she was not able to do. It describes a performance, in the form of an observable behavior, that the learner will be able to achieve and that can be evaluated. According to Mager: "If you don't know where you're going, you run the risk of ending up where you didn't want to be" (2).

Learning objectives provide a framework for teaching. They help structure the learning process and select appropriate learning activities. Finally, they provide a guide for constructing an assessment that is consistent with the objectives and learning activities proposed.

The objective-based approach offers a number of advantages, such as: making pedagogical objectives precisely explicit, being able to monitor learning, aiming for high taxonomic levels through complex activities, enabling the integration of knowledge from different cognitive, psychomotor and affective domains, being able to assess in a measurable way according to docimological perspectives with a multitude of assessment means, and facilitating the planning approach to a learning process (3, 4).

The aim of our pedagogical module is to plan a learning sequence with operational objectives in order to obtain a performance, in the form of an observable and assessable behavior performed by the learner. For each objective, we will specify the learning and assessment methods that could be adapted.

PEDAGOGICAL SCENARIO

1.1. Training needs:

The chosen theme is common to two specialties: physical medicine and occupational medicine. Close collaboration between the occupational physician and the physical physician helps to improve care and prevent the onset of chronicity.

Acute and chronic low back pain is both a public and occupational health problem, with a direct impact on job loss and economic and social benefits (5).

Given that low back pain is also the third leading cause of perceived disability due to various illnesses, the identification of risk factors, particularly in the workplace, would appear to be of great importance for the implementation of suitable prevention programs (6).

Low back pain remains a common condition, with an estimated lifetime prevalence of around 80%. Progression to chronicity (lasting more than 3 months) is observed in 6 to 8% of cases. It should be emphasized that 90% of patients recover within 4 to 6 weeks, while sub-acute low-back pain (between 4-6 weeks and the end of the 3rd month) affects only 3% of patients (7).

In Tunisia, a study of hospital staff at the Fattouma-Bourguiba University Hospital in Monastir showed a cumulative prevalence of low-back pain of 57.1%, an annual prevalence of 50.1% and a prevalence of chronic low-back pain of 12.8% (8). In fact, low-back pain generally has a multifactorial origin, the most recognized risk factors being: overweight and obesity, biomechanical constraints such as manual handling, anteflexion of the trunk associated with twisting or whole-body vibration when driving vehicles, psychosocial factors such as stress at work and repetitive tasks.

The consequences of low back pain are manifold, essentially affecting the health of the worker, ranging from the difficulty of daily tasks due to pain, to the obligation to reclassify, evict and even lose work, as well as early retirement and even surgery. These consequences also affect companies, which suffer enormous financial and economic losses in terms of lost working days, care costs and workers' compensation.

This suggests the importance of raising awareness among occupational health professionals (family doctors, physical physicians, occupational physicians) of the need to recognize this condition, so that it can be managed early and appropriately.

Our theme meets the PUIGER criteria. In particular, because of its high **prevalence**, its **urgent** nature, particularly in the acute forms of the disease, the possibility of effective **intervention** by healthcare structures in its management, notably to prevent the transition to chronic forms resistant to medical treatment, its **exemplary** pedagogical role in the context of adapted treatment, and lastly, its significant social and economic **repercussions**.

The management of common low-back pain in a patient, particularly in the workplace, involves positive diagnosis, assessment of the degree of functional incapacity and therapeutic planning. This is a complex skill to acquire in physical medicine. For residents in occupational medicine, the study of this topic helps them to identify the occupational risk factors for the onset or aggravation of low back pain in a working patient, to assess the patient's medical suitability for the workplace, and to develop hygiene measures to prevent relapses. In addition, for residents in physical medicine and occupational medicine, low back pain is a frequent reason for consultation and a theme included in their post-graduate teaching and end-of-specialty examination.

1.2. Target audience :

The training is designed for future specialists (residents) in physical and occupational medicine at all levels.

1.3. Overall course :

This educational sequence lasts six weeks, one week for each objective. Each resident must validate objectives. For each objective, we have established means of learning and evaluation, while respecting the pedagogical alignment and coherence between them.

1.4. Learning objectives :

For in-depth, sustainable learning, we have chosen learning objectives that cover the 3 domains of knowledge: knowing, knowing how and knowing how to be (Figures n°1 and 2). It's not uncommon for a learning objective to fall under several domains, or even all three. In such cases, it's not a question of classifying it in a single domain at all costs, but rather of determining the one that predominates, or the one we want to emphasize (9,10).
The cognitive domain covers learning in the areas of knowledge, mental and intellectual activities, critical and reflective thinking, and problem-solving.

The psychomotor domain, on the other hand, allows us to report on learning related to know-how, dexterity, professional movements, motor and physical skills.

The social-emotional domain allows us to account for learning related to self-management, social attitudes, interpersonal skills, values and emotional intelligence.

We're aiming for level 2 or 3 depth according to Bloom's taxonomy.

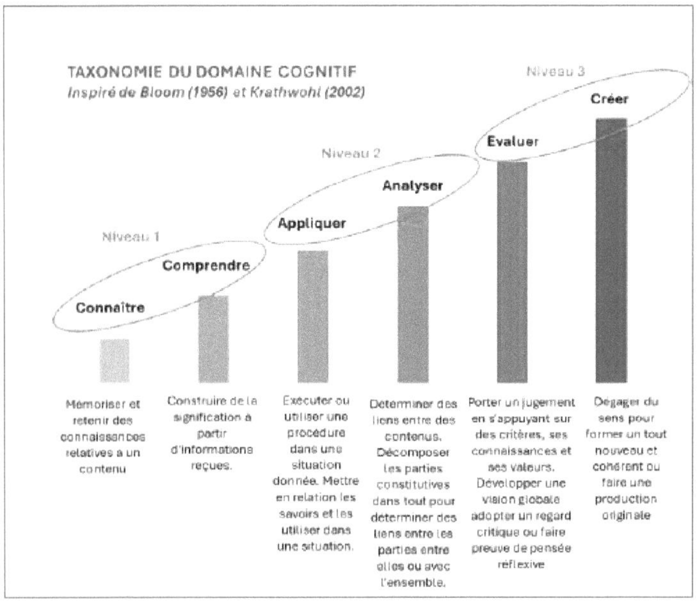

Figure 1: Taxonomy of the cognitive domain (4)

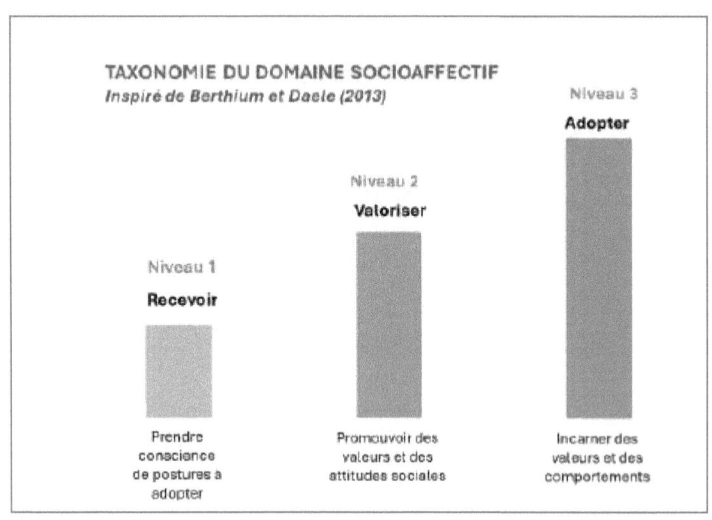

Figure 2: Taxonomy of psychoaffective and psychomotor domains (4)

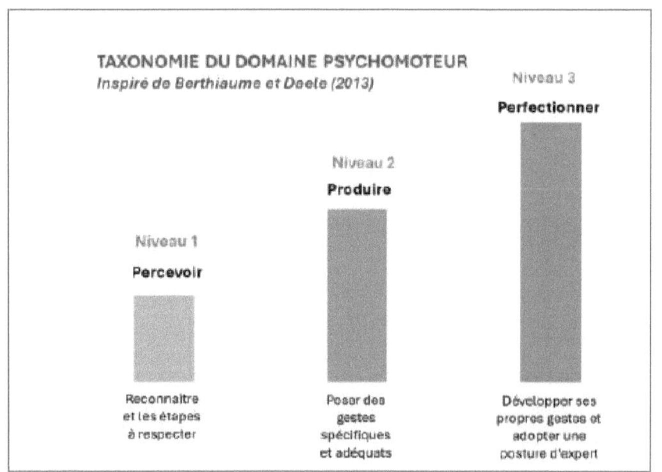

Figure 3: Taxonomy of the psychomotor domain(4)

1.4.1. Cognitive domain objectives :

- Identify risk factors for the onset and chronicity of low back pain in working adults
- Gather anamnestic, clinical and paraclinical evidence in favor of the etiology of low back pain
- Planning multidisciplinary management of chronic low back pain
- Ruling on the medical fitness of a working adult suffering from low back pain

1.4.2. Psychomotor objectives :

- Performing a clinical examination on a patient with low back pain

1.4.3. Psycho-affective objectives :

- Educating workers with low back pain about spinal hygiene measures
The different learning methods are summarized in table n I. °
The spatio-temporal framework of all these means is summarized in a chronological map (figure n°3).

Table I Learning and assessment methods for different objectives

Objective	Level	Learning medium	Means of assessment
Cognitive domain			
Identify risk factors for the onset and chronicity of low back pain in working adults	Cognitive/2	Flipped classroom (Video clips, articles, etc.) Face-to-face session to draw up a summary diagram	Concept map with evaluation grid
Gather anamnestic, clinical and paraclinical evidence in favor of the etiology of low back pain	Cognitive/3	Clinical Reasoning Apprenticeship (CRA)	Objective structured clinical examination (OSCE)
Planning the therapeutic management of low back pain	Cognitive/3	Case Based Learning (CBL)	Clinical cases
Ruling on the medical fitness of a working adult suffering from low back pain	Cognitive /3	Mini self-learning module (MMAA)	Script Concordance Test (SCT)
Psychomotor domain			

Performing a clinical examination on a patient with low back pain	Psychomotor/2	Commented video clip	Clinical supervision at the patient's bedside
Psychoaffective domain			
Educating workers with low back pain about spinal hygiene measures	Psychoaffective /2	Role-playing	ECOS simulated patient station

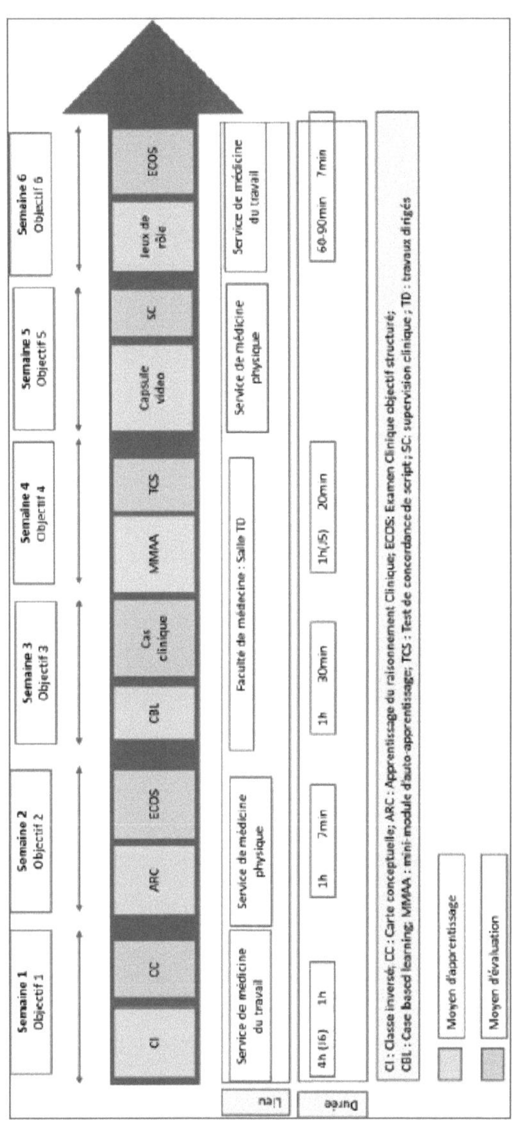

Figure 4: Chronological map of the different learning and assessment methods used

1.5. Learning resources :

A teaching method is defined as the set of principles and theories on which learning activities are based (11).

There are several types of learning methods: affirmative, interrogative, demonstrative and experiential or active. The choice of method depends on the objectives to be achieved, the learner profile and the logistical resources available (12).

1.5.1. The flipped classroom :

The first objective, "to identify the risk factors for the onset and chronicity of low back pain in working adults", is a level 2 cognitive domain learning objective according to Bloom's taxonomy, since the student must be able to identify the risk factors for the onset of low back pain in working adults, and determine the role of some of these factors in the transition to chronicity. The aim is therefore to understand and interpret information. For this purpose, we have chosen the active flipped classroom as a learning medium. To this end, we will provide students with resources (scientific articles, video sequences and practical guides) detailing the etiological factors of low back pain. All these resources will be accessible to learners via useful links.

After explaining the principle, learners are given a week's preparation time to consult the video and read the support materials. After this time, a face-to-face session will enable learners to summarize the etiologies of low back pain, using a diagram that will gradually be drawn up through a group activity. Once the task has been explained, the tutor will act as a discussion guide, emphasizing what is important, creating links between ideas and helping learners to correct any "mistakes". The instructions for the task will specify that the diagram must be in the form of a concept map. A reference diagram is prepared by the tutor to avoid forgetting certain fundamental notions. If necessary, this diagram will be presented to the learners at the end of the session as a summary.

The flipped classroom (FCL) strategy is perfectly suited to an approach that combines face-to-face and distance learning, hence the classic 4-stage flipped classroom (Figure 4): a first stage before the class (outside the classroom), a second stage (in the classroom), a third stage outside the classroom, and a fourth stage to summarize the training (13,14).

- Period 1 (distance learning: outside the classroom): The learner, following the teacher/tutor's instructions, will watch a video, look for information, learn about the theme, bring back elements from the context visited, structure them somewhat, prepare a small presentation in an original way (information search, validation, analysis, synthesis, creativity...).

- Period 2 (face-to-face): In class, in the presence of the teacher, the learner can present the information and resources found, identify differences and spot similarities, experience a socio-cognitive "conflict", clarify preconceptions, raise questions and hypotheses (communication, analysis, reflexivity, modeling...).

- Period 3 (distance): outside the classroom: The learner, outside the classroom and at his or her own pace, can familiarize himself or herself with the theories, identify the elements relevant to the topic under investigation, prepare a synthesis, practice how the model works (learning, making links, memorizing, asking and preparing questions, modeling...).

- Period 4 (face-to-face): Once again in the classroom, the learner, with the help of the teacher, can consolidate what has been learned, make the model or theory work in relation to the themes investigated, prepare for transfer by approaching other situations (understanding, applying, investigating limits, transferring to other contexts...).

Figure 3 summarizes these 4 phases, adapting them to the Kolb cycle. In short, a flipped classroom works by hybridizing two face-to-face sessions and two distance learning sessions outside the classroom. A good understanding of the educational objectives and the learners inevitably requires a scripted approach to learning.

Advantages of the IC strategy include:

- Stimulating the learning of clinical reasoning by verbalizing the thought process;

- Keeping learners alert and motivated;

- Active learning by seeking information;

- The organization of acquired knowledge and its application;

 - And the atmosphere is conducive to communication between learners and trainer.

Thus, the flipped classroom is well suited to learning this cognitive objective, for a limited number of learners accustomed to active learning, such as our residents. However, it is a time-consuming method that cannot be used for a large number of learners (13,14).

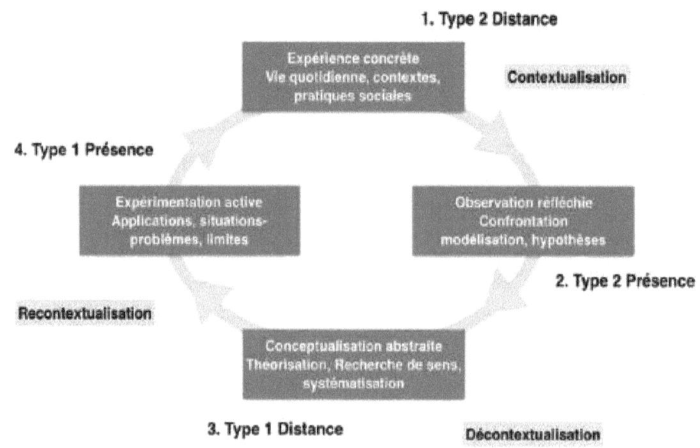

Figure 5: The four phases of the flipped classroom.

1.5.2. Clinical reasoning training (CRT) :

Clinical reasoning (CR) corresponds to the thought processes that enable the clinician to make decisions about the most appropriate actions in a specific health problem-solving context. The specific CRA sessions developed by Chamberland were designed to explicitly involve students in a clinical approach, and to promote the active construction and reorganization of clinical knowledge in students on placement. According to the original method, a clinical situation in the form of a patient's consultation with a doctor is presented to small groups of six to eight students, at their placement site, for 60 to 90 minutes. The students approach a defined problem and pathological entity. With the help of a tutor, they work out the intermediate stages of the CR aloud. They generate diagnostic hypotheses based on the data they gather through questions targeting data from the interview, the clinical examination and the results of various complementary tests. As information is gathered, the hypotheses generated are validated or eliminated, modified or updated, and enriched by new hypotheses. In the end, they arrive at the final diagnosis and draw up the therapeutic plan. The tutor then summarizes the session and decontextualizes it (15). Table II summarizes the various stages of a CRA session.

Table II Steps in an ARC session (15)

1. CONTEXTUALIZATION		
40 minutes	About a predetermined clinical scenario, active data reconstruction: hypothesis generation and evaluation	- Revealing the reason for consultation - Reconstituting clinical data aloud - Reveal out-of-date data, if necessary - Problem formulation - Evaluation of assumptions - Drawing up an investigation plan - Reassess hypotheses and select final diagnosis - Drawing up a treatment plan
2. DECONTEXTUALIZATION/RECONTEXTUALIZATION		
15 minutes	Decontextualization Recontextualization	- Summary : - general approach to the clinical situation - investigation and treatment of the disease entity -Illustration with additional examples
3. EVALUATION OF INDIVIDUAL AND COLLECTIVE LEARNING		
5 minutes		- Self-evaluation of learning -Setting personal learning objectives

This learning method has several advantages: it encourages students to verbalize their thoughts and thus promote clinical reasoning aloud. This will help build confidence, encourage the exchange of ideas between learners and thus enable active learning that keeps learners alert and motivated. CRA also encourages the organization of knowledge. On the other hand, it is time-consuming, applies to a small number of learners and focuses exclusively on clinical reasoning (15).

A pedagogical production of an ARC entitled lombalgie is provided in appendix 1.

1.5.3. Case-Based Learning:

Case-Based Learning (CBL) is a highly topical, active medical learning method that promotes trainer-learner interactivity and enables better integration of knowledge based on a given situation. Case-based learning calls for the study, analysis and interpretation of a given case in order to draw out new knowledge to be integrated according to a hierarchy, and to make it mobilizable in subsequent learning or practice situations. It's a learner-centred learning approach designed to prepare students for clinical practice. This form of learning takes place in small groups of students and a tutor. The group attempts to analyze the problematic arising from the case, using critical reflection strategies (16).

The learner-centered discussion helps to integrate the knowledge gained from the case study. The tutor facilitates group discussion, helping by correcting learners' erroneous assertions and explaining more complex concepts.

CBL learning involves several stages:

- Step 1: The case for the session is presented by the tutor (displayed on a large screen and/or on paper). Learners read and summarize the case.

- Step 2: Students underline key words and clarify terms (documentary research, internet ...)

- Step 3: Students try to propose concepts (key information around which a series of notions and knowledge are organized; these are phenomena that need to be explained and acquired).

- Step 4: Organize concepts into an explanatory diagram, illustrating the links between them: The concept map: This is a graphic illustration of concepts and the links between them as perceived by one or more learners.

- Step 5: Formulate learning objectives.

- Step 6: Acquire relevant information (documentary work, practical work, self-study module, etc.) in relation to the case through individual work.

- Step 7: This is a summing-up step, integrating the newly acquired information; new questions about the case may be raised.

1.5.4. Self-learning mini-module (MMAA) :

The $4^{\text{ème}}$ objective is to decide on the medical aptitude of an adult with low-back pain in the workplace, based on anamnestic, clinical and paraclinical data. This is a level 3 cognitive domain objective. The learning tool we have chosen for this objective is the MMAA.

This pedagogical document presented the theme, the educational objectives, the main pedagogical messages and specified the learners' level of study. A pre-test preceded the pedagogical document and was also used as a post-test. As a result, we chose two clinical cases. The first clinical case included three short open-ended questions (QROC), and the second clinical case included two multiple-choice questions (QCM). The answers were recorded in the basic document provided at the end of the mini-module.

The residents have benefited from a pedagogical device to which they can continually refer in order to progress in their learning process at their own pace. This support has enabled them to stimulate their scientific curiosity with a view to improving their level of learning, and to manage awkward clinical contexts in their daily work. As for the teacher, the advantages of MMAA are manifold. Given that he or she is not always available to supervise residents, the development of such supports enables him or her to fulfil and guarantee his or her task as tutor, even at a distance from the learners.

According to the experiences described in the literature, this active learning method enabled the learner to feel autonomous and to improve his or her level of learning (17). In addition, the learning mini-module offered trainees a transition from theory to practice in a hospital environment, providing them with the opportunity to situate their knowledge, simulate their creativity and self-evaluate. What's more, as medical disciplines in higher education become more comprehensive and precise, the teacher has found himself obliged to develop his teaching devices for the benefit of learners, with a view to ensuring that resident trainees assimilate scientific details and pedagogical messages. Learning through such pedagogical devices has enabled trainees to learn at their own pace, limit their migratory movements to improve their attitudes towards their training, and acquire enthusiasm and self-confidence.

However, trainees may find it difficult to self-evaluate their learning, due in part to the lack of fruitful interaction with the teacher.

1.5.5. Video capsules:

It is well known that the encoding of information is greatly facilitated when this verbal information is coupled with another stimulus, such as a visual stimulus. A CP is defined as a video representation of practices in a given context (18). From a pedagogical point of view, using a video device accelerates comprehension, facilitates memorization, supports attention and structures animation (18, 19). What's more, this approach is appreciated by learners and requires few resources (19, 20). Some authors state that the use of a PC prior to a simulation could reduce the student's perceived anxiety and improve confidence in his or her ability to perform a given task (21, 22).

Adding a CP representing best practices to the simulation could reduce situational anxiety and improve teamwork performance in the context of an emergency situation, a surgical procedure or, as in our case, the practice of a clinical examination on a patient with low back pain (23).

1.5.6. Role-playing: therapeutic education :

The introduction of communication skills training, particularly in doctor-patient communication, is a widespread practice that offers many advantages (24). Among these, the use of the simulated patient provides medical residents with opportunities to practice in situations that mimic what happens in the real world, but in an environment that is safe for the patient, with the possibility of repeating gestures. Training with a simulated patient also enables the scenario to be targeted to exercise specific skills and explore emotionally charged situations. It is now well established that communication between doctor and patient has a major influence on the quality of the doctor-patient relationship. In particular, good doctor-patient communication enhances the effectiveness of the consultation in terms of information gathering, patient understanding of the diagnosis, and patient compliance with treatment.

Role-playing is a teaching method that requires strict adherence to rules, both in the planning stages and in the three phases of the game: before, during and after.

We will organize this teaching session with a simulated patient playing the role of a worker suffering from low back pain. The setting and context of the consultation will be presented by the teacher to all participants beforehand. The clinical vignette has been previously taught to the person who will play the role of the simulated patient, who will also be chosen from among the occupational medicine residents. During the session, a resident will volunteer to conduct the interview with the simulated patient. The aim of the game is to conduct a therapeutic education session with a patient suffering from low back pain, who consults us to return to work. The rest of the group, in the presence of the teacher, follows the interview. The only instruction given to the student playing the doctor's role is to conduct a "normal" consultation, i.e. 15 to 20 minutes. Once the interview is over, the same people meet to discuss each other's impressions, gathering first the comments of the active student, then those of the observers under the direction of the teacher (25).

An example is shown in the appendix (Appendix 2).

1.6. Valuation methods :

Learning is only as good as its assessment. There is a close link between objectives and the evaluation of their achievement. Some have even suggested that learning assessment should be planned immediately after the formulation of objectives. This step is often the most neglected, especially in continuing education.

Yet it is perhaps the most important (26). Evaluation can be either formative or summative.

- Formative assessment means setting out in advance the criteria according to which the required skills will be assessed, formulating them on a form and, above all, giving the student regular feedback on his or her progress. This is done during the module. Giving feedback to students enables pedagogical adjustment (informing the teacher about knowledge acquisition) (27).

  The main aim of formative assessment is to indicate to both teacher and learner the difficulties encountered, so that together they can try to remedy them (28).

- Summative assessment takes place at the end of a module or year. It has an administrative, often sanctioning, evaluation function. For example, it allows students to move on to the next year (27). The aim of summative evaluation is to establish whether learning has been effective (28).

The means of assessment are numerous and polymorphous. The choice of means must be guided by the educational objective pursued and the decisions to be made at the end of the assessment. There is no such thing as a "gold standard" assessment method. An optimal assessment must combine multiple qualitative, quantitative, formative and summative means of evaluation, with constant to-and-fro between simulated contexts and authentic professional practice.

As for the evaluation of the first objective, we opted for the elaboration of a concept map by each resident. An evaluation grid was prepared beforehand.

We have chosen an Objective Structured Clinical Examination (OSCE) and a discussion of a clinical case as the means of assessment for cognitive objectives 2 and 3.

The discussion of a clinical case and the structured objective clinical examination will be used as a summative assessment. We have opted for the TCS for the 4ème objective relating to the elaboration of the decision of medical aptitude for work. The 5ème psychomotor objective is assessed by means of a SC in the patient's bed. The final psycho-affective objective was assessed using a simulated patient ECOS station.

1.6.1. The concept map :

Evaluation of the first objective is carried out individually, by asking each resident to draw a concept map for 15 minutes, using a pre-prepared evaluation grid. This evaluation is followed by a 45-minute in-class feedback session. The concept map is defined by the representation of concepts, the polymorphic links that connect them and the hierarchy of these concepts. This type of tool can be used to assess mental activity during clinical reasoning. It gives an idea of the processes involved in a formative evaluation context, without prejudging results and performance. It can also be used to assess declarative knowledge (29). The use of concept maps as a means of assessment offers a number of advantages, such as the wealth of information gathered, the structuring and hierarchization of concepts assimilated, and the validity of links between different concepts. They fit in well with the assessment of a level 2 cognitive domain objective, with pedagogical alignment with the flipped classroom as a means of learning.

1.6.2. Objective structured clinical examination (OSCE):

It consists in breaking down clinical skills into several sub-skills to be achieved, which become the objective of a workshop or assessment station. The student is then subjected to assessment workshops designed to reproduce the targeted competencies. This assessment method is widely used for semiological skills (medical interview, physical examination, medical reasoning based on the analysis of clinical signs, semiological analysis of a complementary examination, assessment of interpersonal skills, etc.). This method has been proposed as a prototype for the formative assessment of clinical skills, but it poses a problem of construct validity, since it assumes that the sum of the elementary skills represents the final target skill. It is a non-authentic assessment, but richly contextualized.

Evaluation sequences can be of several types:

- Standardized patient station. The student interacts with a standardized patient, i.e. a simulated patient. This may be an actor, an expert patient, a teacher or a former patient who has learned a scenario and been trained.

  The student may be asked to carry out an anamnesis, a clinical examination, a technical procedure, a management procedure, etc. The student is assessed on the performance of this task, as well as on communication, ethical and relational aspects. The student is assessed on task performance, communication, ethical and relational aspects. Debriefing phases may be added at certain stations, to allow the student to explain his or her conduct.

- Station with equipment. The student must perform a procedure, describe or interpret clinical elements. Mannequins, audio or video recordings, photos, anatomical or histological specimens, etc. may be used for this purpose.

Its main advantage lies in its excellent content validity, tempered by its cumbersome organization, which consumes a lot of time for teachers and assessment organizers, especially since, according to the principle of formative assessment, sessions must theoretically be repeated. Its main disadvantage is that it is not entirely consistent with the constructivist paradigm, since it does not address the evaluation of students in complex situations (30).

Two examples are presented in the appendices (appendices 3 and 4) for objectives 2 and 6.

1.6.3. Discussion of a clinical case :

The advantage of this method is that it's active and interactive, enabling better integration of knowledge based on a concrete clinical situation. Its aim is to prepare learners for clinical practice. The clinical vignette is one of the most widely used tools for assessment, in addition to its role in learning, as it provides comprehensive steps where possible etiology, individual patient characteristics, symptoms and signs, family history, important investigations and relevant information are revealed and explained (31). Carolyn Jeffries et al. define vignettes as short, incomplete stories that are written to reflect, in a less complex way, real-life situations in order to encourage discussion and potential solutions to problems where several solutions are possible (32).

It is one of the formats used to assess problem-solving skills and decision-making processes, including clinical judgments made by healthcare professionals, as well as professionalism (33). Kathiresan J, et al (34) stated that the vignette-based discussion method enables learners to apply their clinical reasoning skills in real-life contexts, and that this method motivates them towards self-directed learning and knowledge sharing. In addition, case vignettes are a promising complement to existing means of assessment. Interactive discussion sessions based on clinical vignettes transform residents' approach to patients and their problem-solving and decision-making skills, thereby improving the quality of care.

1.6.4. Script matching tests :

Script concordance tests (SCTs) use short vignettes (describing problematic clinical situations and chosen according to the reasoning to be assessed in the participant) written according to Charlin's recommendations (35,36). Briefly, each vignette presents a short clinical scenario from which several relevant diagnostic or therapeutic hypotheses can be formulated (column 1). Additional information (clinical, biological results, etc.) is then available (column 2), whose relevance to the hypothesis under discussion is assessed on a Likert scale from -2 to +2 (column 3).

The idea is to confront the occupational physician with a complex situation, as close as possible to his or her actual activity. The TCS measures the degree of organization and elaboration of knowledge. It aims to measure the adequacy of links within clinical knowledge, rather than the mere presence of knowledge elements (37).

One of the fundamental advantages of the TCS is that it integrates the context of uncertainty into decision-making, whether diagnostic or therapeutic (38, 39). Assessment of uncertainty or lack of consensus is made possible by the way scores are calculated, using composite scores (38). The principle of such scores is to weight the response and obtain the final score by adding up the scores for each item (40).

Uncertainty management is a common feature of occupational medicine, particularly when diagnosing the occupational origin of a disease, or when deciding on medical fitness for work for a given position, where clinical factors must be compared with occupational factors, and in particular with specific occupational exposure situations (multiple exposure). As such, the TCS is a conceptually attractive means of assessment in occupational medicine and, beyond, in other medical fields. For our residents, we'll be carrying out a TCS in the middle of the internship and a second one before the end of the internship, and we'll be correcting them after the responses have been collected. Each TCS will consist of 5 clinical situations, all independent of each other, each comprising three items, for a total of 15 items.

1.6.5. Direct clinical supervision at the patient's bedside:

This means of assessment is of interest for psychomotor objectives, and promotes an educational culture of self-criticism, focused on patient safety and quality of care (41). Its aim is to monitor the effectiveness and safety of practices. The trainer will observe the learner performing a solo clinical examination on a patient with low-back pain. The trainer will assess the learner's professionalism, time management and skill, using an evaluation grid. He will intervene in the event of difficulties. During the feedback phase following the professional task, the trainer will communicate specific information to the learner based on the observation already made, with the intention of helping him/her improve for future tasks. The disadvantages are the stress and ethical problems associated with the presence of the evaluator, and the cumbersome organization for large groups (42).

<u>CONCLUSION</u>

Low back pain is a frequent complaint. In view of their personal and professional repercussions, it is important to identify their origin in order to provide an appropriate response to the pain. Early positive and etiological diagnosis, as well as therapeutic management, is an integral part of training; hence the interest in designing a pedagogical training project in this area, integrating digital tools in the form of hybrid teaching.

This hybrid training project is adapted to the institutional context in which it will be applied. It has incorporated a range of digital and multimedia teaching resources, and has proposed a variety of distance and/or face-to-face teaching activities with a multidisciplinary approach.

In this work, we have developed a pedagogical project based on the objective-based approach, enabling comprehensive management of a patient consulting for low-back pain. The learning resources chosen, as well as the means of assessment, must provide the learner with a context that resembles that of professional practice, while respecting pedagogical alignment.

However, a number of obstacles discourage the implementation of such projects, notably the time teachers have to devote to mastering, developing and implementing e-learning tools. High costs and a lack of resources and infrastructure also limit the scope for such training.

<u>REFERENCES</u>

1. Kaufman D. Teaching-centered or learner-centered education: a false dichotomy. Pédagogie Médicale, 2002; 3: 145-147.

2. Kahloul N, Ayache H, Azzabi A, Ben Amor H. Les Objectifs pédagogiques (taxonomy, knowledge and their organization). Fame'sview. Bulletin de la faculté de médecine Ibn el Jazzar de Sousse, N°7. 2017

3. Magali MARZO. Formulating learning objectives. Tip sheet. University of Lorraine

4. Nguyen D-Q , Blais J-G. Approche par objectifs ou approche par compétences? Repères conceptuels et implications pour les activités d'enseignement, d'apprentissage et d'évaluation au cours de la formation clinique. Pédagogie Médicale 2007;8:232-51

5. Karine P. Haute Autorité de santé. 2019;178.

6. Vos T, Allen C, Arora M, Barber RM, Bhutta ZA, Brown A, et al. Global, regional, and national incidence, prevalence, and years lived with disability for 310 diseases and injuries, 1990-2015: a systematic analysis for the Global Burden of Disease Study 2015. The Lancet. 8 Oct 2016;388(10053):1545-602.

7. Bontrup C, Taylor WR, Fliesser M, Visscher R, Green T, Wippert PM, et al. Low back pain and its relationship with sitting behaviour among sedentary office workers. Appl Ergon. 1 Nov 2019;81:102894.

8. Bejia I, Younes M, Hadj Belgacem J, Khalfallah T, Ben Salem K, Touzi M, et al. Prevalence and factors associated with common low back pain in hospital staff. Rev Rhum. May 1, 2005;72(5):427-32.

9. Herling, F. (2019). Targeting and formulating learning objectives, pedagogical nudge. [online] Direction de l'apprentissage et de l'innovation pédagogique, HEC Montréal. Available at:

https://ernest.hec.ca/video/DAIP/pdf/Coup_de_Pouce_Pedagogique_ 1_ Cibler_et_formuler_des_objectifs_d_apprentissage.pdf

10. Krathwohl. DR..A Revision of Bloom's Taxonomy: An Overview. https://www.depauw.edu/files/resources/krathwohl.pdf

11. Jean P. Pour une planification méthodoque des activités de formation. Pédagogie Médicale.2001; 2(2) :101-7

12. Sousa M , Mari R. Echange sur les méthodes pédagogiques et techniques d'animation. Sources: L'Oréal teachers' seminar.

13. S. MOUGOU, A. MTIRAOUI. The flipped classroom: The philosophy of a learning method through lived experience. Fame's view. Bulletin de la faculté de médecine Ibn el Jazzar de Sousse, N°7. 2017

14. Lebrun M, The school of tomorrow: between MOOC and flipped classroom n° 156 - June 2015 - 45.

15. Martine Chamberland, M.D., F.R.C.P.C., M.Ed., Dipl. 3e cycle (Ped. Univ.) Les séances d'apprentissage du raisonnement clinique (ARC) : description de la méthode pédagogique. Faculty of Medicine and Health Sciences. Revision : March 26, 2007

16. Chunhua Ma, Wei Zhou. Effects of unfolding case-based learning on academic achievement, critical thinking, and self-confidence in undergraduate nursing students learning health assessment skills. Nurse Education in Practice, 8 March 2022.

17. Deslauriers L, McCarty LS, Miller K, Callaghan K, Kestin G. Measuring actual learning versus feeling of learning in response to being actively engaged in the classroom. Proc Natl Acad Sci U S A. 24 Sep 2019;116(39):19251-7.

18. Kaamouchi NEL, Ann UCA. White paper to help design educational video vignettes.2019

19. Peraya D. At the heart of Mooc, video capsules: a revival of educational television? Distances et médiations des savoirs, 17.2017.

20. Manea AR. La capsule vidéo " moyen de transfert " de la connaissance en FLE d'une situation A à A n+1 situations- chausser de nouvelles lunettes sur le monde à l'ère du numérique - (1) : 1-15.

21. Coyne E, Frommolt V, Rands H, Kain V, Mitchell M. Simulation videos presented in a blended learning platform to improve Australian nursing students' knowledge of family assessment. Nurse Educ Today [Internet]. 2018 ;66 :96-102. Available from: https://doi.org/10.1016/j.nedt.2018.04.012)

22. Tyerman J, Luctkar-Flude M, Graham L, Coffey S, Olsen-Lynch E. A Systematic Review of Health Care Presimulationn Preparation and Briefing Effectiveness. ClinSimulNurs [Internet]. 2019;27:12-25.Available from: https://doi.org/10.1016/j.ecns.2018.11.002).

23. Ledoux, I., Vincelette, C., Lavoie, S., Marceau, M., Bilodeau, C., and Gosselin E. Integration of an educational vignette into the briefing of nursing students in an emergency care simulation context: acceptability and effects on situational anxiety and teamwork. SciNurs Heal PractInfirm Prat en santé. 2019 ;2(2) :1-13

24. Humphris GM, Kaney S. Assessing the development of communication skills in undergraduate medical students. Medical education. 2001;35(3):225-31

25. Girard G, Clavet D, Boulé R. Planning and facilitating a role-playing game beneficial to learning. Pédagogie Médicale. August 1, 2005;6(3):178-85.

26. Jean P . Pour une planification méthodoque des activités de formation. Pédagogie Médicale.2001 ; 2(2) :101-7) double.

27. Barrier JH, Brazeau-Lamontagne L, Colin R, Quinton A, Liorca G, Ehua FS. Professionalism training for future physicians. Recommandations du conseil Pédagogique de la CIDMEF. Pédagogie Médicale. 2004 ;5(2) :75-81.

28. Giordan André. L'enseignement scientifique : comment faire pour que " ça marche " ? In : Paris : Delagrave.2002

29. A short guide to medical education & clinical evaluation. Collège national enseignants odontologie conservatrice. September 2011

30. Guilbert J-J. Guide pédagogique pour les personnels de santé, Sixième édition. 1990 ;392

31. Depaigne-Loth A, Rullon I M V. Vignettes cliniques Ŕ Exercer et évaluer ses prises de décision. Risques Qual. 2021;18(2):91Ŕ6.

32. Jeffries C, Maeder DW. Using vignettes to build and assess teacher understanding of instructional strategies. Professional Educator. 2005;27(1 & 2):17Ŕ28.

33. Nendaz MR, Raetzo MR, Junod AF, Vu NV. Teaching diagnostic skills: clinical vignette or chief complaints? Adv Health Sci Educ. 2000;5:3Ŕ10.

34. Kathiresan J, Patro BK. Case vignette: a promising complement to clinical case presentations in teaching. EducHealth. 2013;26:21Ŕ24

35. Charlin B, Roy L, Brailovsky C, Goulet F, van der Vleuten C. The Script Concordance test: a tool to assess the reflective clinician. Teaching and learning in medicine. 2000;12(4):189-95

36. Charlin B, Gagnon R, Sibert L, Van der Vleuten C. The script concordance test, an instrument for assessing clinical reasoning. Pédagogie médicale. 2002;3(3):135-44.

37. Jouquan J, Bail P. What are we committing to by switching from the teaching paradigm to the learning paradigm? Pédagogie médicale. 2003;4(3):163-75.

38. Charlin B, Desaulniers M, Gagnon R, Blouin D, Van Der Vleuten C. Comparison of an aggregate scoring method with a consensus scoring method in a measure of clinical reasoning capacity. Teaching and learning in medicine. 2002;14(3):150-6.

39. Charlin B, van der Vleuten C. Standardized assessment of reasoning in contexts of uncertainty: the script concordance approach. Evaluation & the health professions. 2004;27(3):304-19.

40. Norcini JJ, Shea JA, Day SC. The use of aggregate scoring for a recertifying examination. Evaluation & the Health Professions. 1990;13(2):241-51.

41. Tomlinson J. Using clinical supervision to improve the quality and safety of patient care: a response to Berwick and Francis. BMC Medical Education 2015; 15:103

42. Laboux O, Pottier P, Renard E. Petit guide de pédagogie médicale et évaluation clinique. 2011 ; Availablefrom: http://www.cneoc.eu/jcneoc/files/Petit Guide de Pédagogie Médicale et Evaluation Clinique. Pdf

APPENDICES

Appendix 1: ARC session (objective no. 2)
Guide du Moniteur

<u>Complaint:</u> low back pain in a 45-year-old man

<u>Objectives :</u>

1. List the diagnoses to be considered in the presence of low back pain, depending on the patient's condition.
2. Gather data from the interview and physical examination to investigate low back pain in relation to the diagnoses evoked
3. Prioritize complementary tests according to the probability of each diagnosis.

<u>Diagnosis to be considered at this stage:</u>

1) Common lumbago of disc origin
2) Posterior inter-apophyseal osteoarthritis
3) Maigne dorsolumbar hinge syndrome
4) Spondylolisthesis
5) Spinal deformity
6) Narrowed lumbar canal
7) Infectious spondylodiscitis
8) Spondyloarthropathy
9) Multiple myeloma or lymphoma
10) Bone metastasis
11) Fractured vertebrae

12) Lumbago of urological origin
13) Digestive (pancreatic) lumbago

Interrogation :

1) <u>History:</u>

- Personal lumbago: in favour of a discal origin
- Personal lumbar trauma, polyarthrosis, physical work involving torsion and anteflexion of the trunk: in favour of a common mechanical origin
- Personal cancer: in favor of spinal bone metastasis

- Family history of ankylosing spondylitis or spondyloarthropathy: in favor of spondyloarthropathy
- Family history of psoriasis: in favor of spondyloarthropathy
- Personal history of psoriasis, inflammatory colopathy (Crohn's disease and ulcerative colitis), peripheral arthritis, sausage toe or finger, talalgia, anterior uveitis: in favour of spondyloarthropathy
- Personnel with recent infection: in favour of infectious spondylodiscitis
- Sports personnel (gymnastics at an early age): in favour of spondylolisthesis
- Personal hematologic malignancy: in favor of low back pain secondary to multiple myeloma or lymphoma
- Early menopause, prolonged amenorrhea, prolonged immobilization, hyperthyroidism or hyperparathyroidism, long-term corticosteroid therapy, fracture: in favour of vertebral compression.
- Familial osteoporosis: in favour of vertebral compression
- Personal or family history of urological pathology (kidney tumour, urinary lithiasis, retroperitoneal fibrosis): in favour of urological low back pain

- Pancreatic tumor or upper rectal tumor patients: in favor of low back pain of digestive origin

2) <u>Characteristic of pain :</u>
   - Mode of onset and evolution :
     - Sudden onset following heavy lifting: in favour of discal origin
     - Sudden onset following a false movement: in favour of posterior inter-apophyseal osteoarthritis
     - Sudden onset following trauma: in favour of vertebral compression
     - Progressive worsening: in favor of a secondary origin
     - Relapse course: in favor of spondyloarthropathy
   - Location and radiation :
     - Low, bilateral or rod-shaped lumbar pain: in favour of disc origin
     - Unilateral low back pain: in favour of posterior inter-apophyseal osteoarthritis
     - Low back or lumbar pain: in favour of vertebral compression
     - Lumbosacral or lumbo-gluteal pain with unilateral pain in the inguinal or pubic region and at the hip: in favor of Maigne's dorsolumbar hinge syndrome
     - Abrupt, acute lumbar pain radiating downwards to the external genitalia: in favour of urological low-back pain
   - Type of pain
     - Mechanical: in favour of a common spinal origin
     - Improved by dorsal decubitus and rest and aggravated by activity and prolonged sitting or standing or carrying of objects: in favour of disc origin

- Inflammatory, especially at night, morning stiffness, does not improve with usual analgesics: in favour of symptomatic low back pain
- Cough, coughing impulse/defecation effort: in favour of disc origin
- Vague discomfort: in favor of Maigne's dorsolumbar hinge syndrome
- Improvement by bending forward and worsening by walking in favour of narrowed lumbar canal.

3) <u>Accompanying signs :</u>
- General signs: fever with chills, sweating, depression: in favor of infectious origin
- The existence of an entry point +++ particularly surgical: in favour of infectious origin
- Diabetes, chronic alcoholism, immunodepression, history of tuberculosis: in favor of infectious origin.
- Altered general condition: in favor of metastatic origin or digestive or urological cancer
- Digestive signs such as nausea, vomiting and transfixing epigastric pain: in favor of chronic pancreatitis
- Sacroiliac pain: gluteal dl, pseudo sciatica with tilt (dl support, tripod), peripheral enthesopathies such as inferior or posterior talalgia; inflammatory anterior thoracic or sausage toe or finger: in favour of APS.
- Extra-articular signs such as diarrhea: in favor of IBD
- Extra-articular signs such as psoriasis and uveitis

RECAP

At this stage, the patient is a 45-year-old man with no previous pathological history of note, who presents with low-back pain following the effort of carrying a heavy load, improved by rest and aggravated by prolonged standing and sitting, with no other associated signs.

Diagnosis unlikely at this stage:

1) Infectious spondylodiscitis
2) Spondyloarthropathy
3) Multiple myeloma or lymphoma
4) Bone metastasis
5) Fractured vertebrae
6) Lumbago of urological origin
7) Digestive (pancreatic) lumbago

Diagnosis to be considered at this stage:

1) Common lumbago of disc origin
2) Posterior inter-apophyseal osteoarthritis
3) Maigne dorsolumbar hinge syndrome
4) Spondylolisthesis
5) Spinal deformity
6) Narrowed lumbar canal

Physical examination :

1) Examination of the static spine :

Painful attitude, segmental paravertebral muscle contracture: points to a disc origin

ILMI can explain low back pain

2) <u>Examination of the dynamic spine :</u>

A fracture sign points to a disc origin

3) <u>Palpatory segmental examination :</u>

Paravertebral pain point at D12-L1, accentuation of ridge pain on pressure, cellulalgia on palpation between painful junction and ridge: point to Maigne syndrome.

RECAP

At this stage, the patient is a 45-year-old man with no previous pathological history of note, who presents with low-back pain following the effort of carrying a heavy load, improved by rest and aggravated by prolonged standing and sitting, with no other associated signs.

On examination, he showed lumbar paravertebral muscle contracture. The examination was otherwise normal.

The most likely diagnosis at this stage:

The most likely diagnosis is low back pain of disc origin.

However, other etiologies of common low back pain remain possible.

Only Maigne's syndrome can be ruled out, given the normality of the palpatory segmental examination.

The patient received the appropriate treatment for the required duration without any improvement. An X-ray of the lumbar spine from the front (Desèze cliché) and from the side was therefore taken.

Additional tests :

<u>RX Standards :</u>

Demineralization in favour of osteoporosis

Transitional anomalies

Spinal statics, scoliosis

Spondylolisthesis on isthmic lysis or isthmic agenesis

Disc pinching, osteophytes, subchondral sclerosis in favor of discarthrosis

Lateral or posterior yawning in favor of soft disc herniation

Posterior inter-apophyseal osteoarthritis

No bone lysis or condensation

 In favour of a narrow lumbar canal: on frontal views: Sagittalization or excessive visibility of posterior joint spaces on at least 3 levels, and inter-pedicular space does not increase from top to bottom on lateral views: Disappearance of the inter-apophyso-lamar rhombus; Sagittalization of joint masses; Shortness of pedicles.

EXPLORATION RESULTS :

Pinched disc

Otherwise clear

Diagnosis : Common lumbago of disc origin

Patient guide

<u>Complaint:</u> low back pain

<u>Interrogation</u> :

A 45-year-old man, with no notable pathological history, consulted for low back pain following the effort of carrying a heavy load, improved by rest and aggravated by prolonged standing and sitting, with no other associated signs.

<u>Physical examination :</u>

On examination, he showed lumbar paravertebral muscle contracture. The examination was otherwise normal.

<u>Further tests</u>

Disc impingement on X-ray

Otherwise clear

Appendix 2: Role-playing (Objective 6)

Scenario title	Educating a worker with low back pain about spinal hygiene measures
Target audience	Future specialists in occupational or physical medicine
Trainer/learner ratio	1/8
Maximum number of learners	8
Frame	x Resident pre-graduate training □ DPC
Protagonists	residents in occupational medicine and physical medicine

1. Pedagogical objectives

1.1 General objective :	- Therapeutic education for workers with chronic low back pain
1.2 Specific objectives:	- Assessing the functional incapacity of a worker with low back pain through history-taking - Identify the professional and psychological factors that contribute to the persistence of low back pain - Educating workers with chronic low back pain about spinal hygiene measures

2. Preparation

2.1 Type of role-playing game	Cognitive (know-how) □ Psycho-affective (interpersonal skills) X Mixed
2.2 Role-playing modality	**Single scene :** Simple[1] □ x Simple with assistant[2] □ Simple inversion follow-up[3] □ Single relay X[4] **Multiple scenes :** Single simultaneous[5] □ Simultaneous rotation[6] □
2.3 Equipment required in the simulation room	Audio-visual equipment x Observation grids x Evaluation grids □ Other ....
2.4. Medical and para-clinical records to be supplied	Paper file: □ Para-clinical elements: □ If yes type:... ....
2.5. Preparin	Session venues: x Occupational medicine department □ in-situ Room set-up: as for a medical consultation..........

| g the room | Others..
 .... |
| | |

[1]:one participant plays the doctor, one the patient, the rest of the group: observers
[2] a doctor, a patient, a physician's assistant
[3] a doctor and a patient switch roles
[4] a few participants take over the role of doctor
[5] participants play all three roles in the trio simultaneously
[6] participants take turns playing the three roles in the trio

3. Simulation session :

- ➢ Session duration: 60-90 minutes

- ➢ Protagonists:

- ➢ Role-playing scenario :

- One participant plays the role of a worker suffering from low back pain. He or she will receive an information sheet with further instructions on the steps to follow.
- A participant will play the role of an occupational physician educating a worker with low back pain.

<u>Starting scenario for the patient :</u>

- You are Mr Ali, aged 50, operator of a semolina bagging line (unit weight of bags: 50 kg) and father of two children.
- You enter the consultation cubicle: you limp as you walk.
- You are a smoker: 1 pack a day for about ten years.
- You seem irritable and anxious, dreading this return to activity.
- You are being seen for a return visit after 25 days' sick leave following a bout of low back pain.
- <u>Only give the following details if the doctor asks you to:</u>
- You've already had a history of low back pain for years, following an accident at work 10 years ago (shortly after you were hired): lumbago following the carrying of heavy loads.
- The accident was not declared for fear of dismissal

- The last attack of low back pain was 2 weeks ago, prompting the patient to consult his rheumatologist.
- During this latest attack of low back pain, you describe low back pain
- You were on extended rest (25 days): the pain was incapacitating, requiring a strict 10-day rest period, extended by 15 days given the persistence of the pain.
- Have you ever been off work for low back pain?
- You have not followed the physical re-education sessions
- You have increasingly reduced activities, with a marked decrease in activities of daily living since the onset of pain.
- You report dissatisfaction with working conditions
- You are certain that your current position is harmful to your health
- You're also certain that the pain is indicative of a serious injury
- You expected the pain to disappear before returning to work, but this was not the case. You fear that the pain will increase with the return to work.
- You report a lack of workplace support from line management
- You complain about working conditions: lifting loads for more than half the day, non-automated work processes
- You request a transfer to a less demanding position, in particular that of a janitor.

<u>Starting scenario for the doctor:</u>

You are an occupational physician in an autonomous medical department.

A worker on sick leave following a bout of low back pain came to see you for a return visit.

This is a worker on the semolina bagging line. He loads the cart with 50 kg bags.

You have already ruled on the patient's suitability for the current position, taking into account the clinical and paraclinical data of the case: transfer to another position for a period of 3 months for temporary incapacity.
You need to educate the patient about spinal hygiene.

3.1 Pre-game briefing :

<u>Instructions for trainers :</u>

- The facilitator explains the process and the objective of the session, and the rules of the game (stressing to the protagonists that they will be playing a role (and not their own function)).
- Explain role-playing, its type and modalities
- Explain the observers' task and provide the grids (observation and/or evaluation)
- Set the duration of jeu□□.
- Explain the progression of play and acquisitions. The last games will benefit from the first and will probably be better. This rule should only be said after the first game.
- Prepare, secure and reassure the protagonists:
  - Creating a climate of trust
  - Confidentiality of exchanges.
  - Freedom to play or not to play, freedom to say or not to say.
  - Explain that this is fiction.
  - Respect for the actors, silence during the performance, no value judgments.

3.2. Procedure :

Expected duration: 20 mn

<u>**Instructions for trainers**</u>

- Choose the different actors on a voluntary basis. The student who will play the role of the patient is given the scenario for the situation.
- Presenting the scenario
- Bring in the actors, announce that the game will last 15 minutes and start playing.
- Make a note of the strong points and remarks that you can then rephrase to relaunch the debate or redirect it towards the session's objectives.
- Stop the game after 15 minutes. It's possible to let the game run over for 1 or 2 minutes if the objective of the session is achieved; announce this then.
- Intervene and, if necessary, stop the game if a player is in difficulty.
- Indicate the end of the game
- At the end of the game: applaud the actors, thank them.

3.3. Debriefing (after the game)

<u>**Instructions for trainers**</u>

- Debrief the protagonists first (self-evaluation)
- Then gather comments from observers (hetero-evaluation)
- Start with the positives
- Accept no value judgments
- Make your comments, you'll be the last to speak
- If the game has been filmed, watch the video and select the interesting parts.

Describe the descriptive phase

Expected duration: 10 mn

- Review defined objectives.

- Discuss the content and conduct of the debriefing session.

- Setting the tone for a respectful environment.

- Answer learners' questions.

- Formulate simple, open-ended questions:

  - What happened?

  - How do you think the role-playing went?

  - How do you feel about your participation?

  - did you enjoy your participation?

  - do you feel like you're taking part in a real consultation?

  - do you find it difficult to play your character?

  - How could you have been more efficient?

  - Did anything make you feel uncomfortable (being observed, being filmed, reviewing the sequence as a group)?

  - What emotions did this experience trigger for you?

  - What was the most difficult moment for you?

Describe the analytical phase

- Expected duration: 10 mn

  - Prepare a list of ideas to be discussed

  - Let participants propose their own interpretations and add to the list of overlooked points.

  - Provide additional information and correct errors

  - Identify best practices

  - Provide examples of good interactions.

  - Discuss how this can be translated into patient care. (*generalize)*

  - Extend the analysis phase with hypotheses (what if...)

Recontextualization: If the patient insists on a professional reclassification?

<u>**Describe the synthesis phase**</u>

- Expected duration: 10mn

- Review what you've learned.

- Ask participants what they would do now if the same situation arose.

"If you had it to do over again, what would you keep? What would you change in your behavior?"

-Give learners feedback on the session as a whole.

- Thank learners for their participation.

4. Precise bibliographical references

(A paper or computer copy of each reference must be supplied with the scenario)

Observation grid :

	Fact	Not done
The doctor makes contact - Greet the patient - Introducing yourself - Home - Listen to the first words without interruption - Explains the reason for consultation		
The interview focuses on the patient, the physician - Uses reformulation (takes up the patient's words and rephrases them) - Uses the patient's words to guide the interview - Ask open-ended questions - Ask targeted semi-open questions: Who? Who? Who? - Clarifies and summarizes (synthesis)		
The doctor identifies and takes into account the patient's non-verbal behavior (anxiety, sighing, crying, etc.).		
Search for F and P history (M/CH/PSY...) and professional history (history of work-related injuries, particularly lumbar trauma).		
Identify risk factors for not returning to work due to illness : History of low back pain Duration of low back pain Severity of pain Severity of functional disability Presence of sciatica Previous work stoppage for low back pain Previous lumbar surgery Strict rest prescription > 7 days		
Evaluate pain and functional disability reported by the patient (pain scale out of 10)		
Removing professional obstacles to recidivism and non-return to work: - Job satisfaction - Perceived relationship between work and back pain - Support from the workplace - Work history		
Exploring the representations he has of his illness in relation to back pain		
The doctor has drawn up advice for therapeutic education: Explain to the patient that he/she must save and protect the spine by gradually learning the correct gestures and attitudes in three areas: -The load handling method -Pure ergonomics in everyday hygiene The doctor has communicated understandable information to the patient about his illness:		
The doctor concludes the interview by planning the next steps: - Explain the fitness decision to the patient, which is a transfer to another position for a period of 3 months due to temporary incapacity. - Periodic re-evaluation of suitability according to clinical evolution - Emphasize multidisciplinary care for better pain control and management - Explain to the patient that he/she should align with the therapeutic plan to improve functional capabilities -Treat any psychological disorders - Social and professional reintegration		
Monitor patient compliance with the therapeutic plan proposed by the attending physician		

| Explain the need for good compliance with back hygiene and the therapeutic plan proposed by the attending physician. | | |

Appendix 3: ECOS station (objective n 2)

ECOS station

<table>
<tr><td>Background :</td><td>Physical medicine consultation</td></tr>
<tr><td>System :</td><td>Locomotor</td></tr>
<tr><td>Complaint:</td><td>Lumbago</td></tr>
</table>

Clinical situation:

A 60-year-old man comes to the clinic with low back pain.

Instructions to the candidate :

You have 7 minutes to :

1- Focused questioning

2- Describe aloud the elements of the clinical examination to look for (you don't have to perform the physical examination; the examination data will be provided by the patient).

3- Request any additional tests required

4- Announcing the most likely diagnosis to the patient

5- Planning what to do

Instructions to the observer :
Please tick done or not done for each ITEM in the corresponding box.

If after 3 minutes the candidate does not begin the clinical examination, you signal to the simulated patient (discreet and defined before the test) to say "you are going to examine me".

If after 5 minutes the candidate does not announce the diagnosis, you signal to the simulated patient (discreet and defined before the test) to say "you're going to prescribe radiological X-rays".

If, after 6 minutes, the candidate still hasn't announced the diagnosis or treatment, signal to the simulated patient (discreet and defined before the test) to say ("Doctor, what's my diagnosis?") and then ("How are you going to treat me?").

If the candidate requests a prostate biopsy with complementary examinations, you will check off what is done in the CAT section.

<table>
<tr><td>

Simulated patient scenario :
You only answer the questions asked
If the condidate asks you if you have any other signs, you ask him or her what type of
    doctor they are.
If the candidate proceeds to complementary examinations without asking about urinary
    signs, you tell him doctor, I forgot to tell you that I have hematuria and pollakiuria.

</td></tr>
<tr><td>

You are Mr H.A., 60 years old, consulting you for low back pain.
You are a worker
Non-smoker
Pain :
Medium intensity, gradually increasing, not improving
Lumbar seat (whole spine, not lower lumbar)
Without irradiation
Onset 6 months ago with no triggering factor
Exacerbation at night: pain wakes you up and is not triggered by a change of position
No history of similar episode or lumbago
No clear improvement with analgesics and anti-inflammatories
No personal history
Family history of cancer death (treated in urology)

</td></tr>
<tr><td>

Presence of hematuria and sometimes pollakiuria
No urinary incontinence, urgency or dysuria
No cough
No swallowing problems
10 kg weight loss in the last 6 months with anorexia
Review:
Dynamic examination of the spine: stiffness (reduced mobility) in all movements
Increased finger-to-ground distance
Shober to 3
No lumbar Lasègue
No hamstring retraction
No motor deficit
No sensitivity disorders
ROTS present and symmetrical
Normal neuroperineal examination

</td></tr>
</table>

Free ganglion areas
TR 40g prostate with suspicious nodule on right with soft bladder floor
Normal thyroid examination
Normal pulmonary auscultation

If the candidate tells you he's going to ask you for spinal X-rays, you say "which ones" if he doesn't specify "face and profile". Then you tell him I've done it and here's the conclusion, and you give him the X-ray report.

If he asks for any additional tests you have available, you give them to him. After 3 minutes, if the observer gives you a sign (discreet and defined before the test), you say to the candidate, "Are you going to examine me, Doctor?

After 5 minutes, if the o observer gives you a sign (discreet and defined before the test), you tell the candidate you're going to ask me for further tests. After 6 minutes, if the observer gives you a sign (discreet and defined before the test), you say ("Doctor, what is my diagnosis?") and add ("How are you going to treat me?").

Observation grid

Items		Fact	Not done
Interrogation			
1	Profession		
2	Pain onset date		
3	Character (timing of exacerbation or morning wake-up call)		
4	Intensity		
5	Evolution		
6	Seat or irradiation		
7	History of low back pain or lumbago		
8	Sedation with analgesics		
9	Medical, surgical or family **history**		
10	Smoking		
11	paraesthesia or paresis or urinary urgency or urinary incontinence due to urinary urgency		
12	**General signs** (asthenia or anorexia or weight loss)		
13	Urinary disorders (hematuria or pollakiuria)		
14	Throat lump or swallowing difficulty		
15	Cough		
Clinical examination			
16	**Dynamic study of the lumbar spine** Flexion or extension or laterality		
17	Finger-to-ground distance		
18	Schober index		
19	Lumbar Lasègue		
20	hamstring retraction		

21	**Neurological examination**: study of motor skills or sensitivity or ROT or neuroperineal examination		
22	Ganglion areas		
23	TR		
24	Ex thyroid		
25	Pulmonary auscultation		
Further tests			
26	VS		
27	**Rx lumbar spine** Face or DESEZE incidence		
28	**Rx lumbar spine** Profile		
29	PSA		
30	Reno-vesicoprostatic or prostatic ultrasound		
Diagnosis			
31	Secondary lumbago		
32	of probable tumor origin (or bone metastasis)		
33	Probable prostate cancer		
CAT			
34	Referral for urology consultation		
35	Endorectal biopsy		

<h1 style="text-align:center"><u>Weighting grid</u></h1>

Items		Pond.
Interrogation		35
1	Profession	1
2	Pain onset date	2
3	Character (timing of exacerbation or morning wake-up call)	4
4	Intensity	2
5	Evolution	3
6	Seat or irradiation	3
7	History of low back pain or lumbago	4
8	Sedation with analgesics	1
9	Mdc or chgi **history**	4
10	Smoking	1
11	paraesthesia or paresis or urinary urgency or urinary incontinence due to urinary urgency	3
12	**General signs** (Asthenia or anorexia or weight loss)	4
13	Urinary disorders (hematuria or pollakiuria)	1
14	Throat lump or swallowing difficulty	1
15	Cough	1
Clinical examination		26
16	**Dynamic study of the lumbar spine** Flexion or extension or laterality	4
17	Finger-to-ground distance	3

18	Schober index	4
19	Lumbar Lasègue	2
20	Retraction IJ	2
21	**Neurological examination**: study of motor skills or sensitivity or ROT or neuroperineal examination	4
22	Ganglion areas	1
23	TR	4
24	Ex thyroid	1
25	Pulmonary auscultation	1
Further tests		19
26	**VS**	4
27	**Lumbar Rx** Face	4
28	**Lumbar Rx** Profile	4
29	PSA	4
30	Reno-vesicoprostatic or prostatic ultrasound	3
Diagnosis		12
31	Secondary lumbago	4
32	of probable tumor origin (or bone metastasis)	4
33	Probable prostate cancer	4
CAT		8

| 34 | Referral for urology consultation | 5 |
| 35 | Endorectal biopsy | 3 |

Appendix 4: ECOS station (objective no. 6)

ECOS station

Level :	Occupational medicine and physical medicine residents
Background :	Consultation
System :	Locomotor
Complaint:	Lumbago

Clinical situation:

Mr M.B, aged 45, a truck driver with 18 years' experience in a freight transport company, is consulting us for a return visit.

Taking into account the clinical and paraclinical data, as well as the patient's workstation study, he has been deemed fit for work, subject to adaptation of his workstation. If necessary, he should be assigned to a workstation that avoids heavy loads and whole-body vibration transmitted by the seat.

Instructions to the candidate :

You have 7 minutes to :

6- Carry out targeted questioning to identify any professional anamnestic factors aggravating the patient's symptomatology.

7- Announcing the fitness decision to the patient

8- Patient education on spinal hygiene measures in the workplace

Instructions to the observer :

Please tick done or not done for each ITEM in the corresponding box.

If after **2**minutes the candidate does not begin the examination, you signal to the simulated patient (discreet and defined before the test) to say "**you are going to examine me**".

If after 4 minutes the candidate does not announce the decision of aptitude, you give a sign to the simulated patient (discreet and defined before the test) so that he says "you are going to change my workstation".

If after 6 minutes the candidate has not begun the therapeutic education, give the simulated patient a sign (discreet and defined before the test) to say "Doctor, what should I do to avoid aggravating my low back pain through work?".

Simulated patient scenario :
You are Mr Mourad, 45 years old,
You have been a truck driver with a freight transport company for 18 years.
No personal history
Smoker 2 packs a day
Pain: Moderate intensity without radiation, occurring at the end of the day, more pronounced on long-distance journeys and calmed by rest.
Onset 3 years ago aggravated by professional driving
You report an exacerbation of low back pain due to long journeys (uncomfortable seat that transmits shocks), carrying heavy loads (boxes of goods) and prolonged sitting.
You are taking a treatment based on analgesics and anti-inflammatories
You fear a recurrence of pain when you return to work
You are requesting a ban on professional driving

<u>Observation grid</u>

Items		Fact	Not done
Interrogation			
	The doctor makes contact: greeting the patient		
	Profession		
	Length of service		
	History		
	Habits		
	Character of pain		
	Gathering patient complaints: factors aggravating pain in the workplace		
Announcing the fitness decision to the patient			
	Write the fitness decision in the worker's fitness sheet		
	Explain the fitness advice to the patient: He is able to do so by arranging his workstation in such a way as to avoid jolting and prolonged sitting in a non-ergonomic position (including the seat): by allowing him short rest periods (10 minutes every two hours) during which he can relax and loosen his back muscles. If necessary, he should be assigned to a workstation that avoids heavy loads and whole-body vibrations transmitted by the seat.		
Patient education			
	Regular, long-term physical exercise and spinal conservation techniques		
	Resuming physical activity and a socio-professional life without apprehension		
	Take 15-minute breaks every two hours (when traveling), during which he can relax and loosen his back muscles.		
	Frequent changes in posture		
	Avoid prolonged sitting		
	Show the patient how to handle loads ergonomically		

<u>Weighting grid</u>

Items		Weighting
Interrogation		**20**
	The doctor makes contact: greeting the patient	1
	Profession	2
	Length of service	2
	History and habits	5
	Character of pain	5
	Gathering patient complaints: factors aggravating pain in the workplace	5
Announcing the fitness decision to the patient		**20**
	Write the decision on suitability on the suitability form and sign it.	5
	Issuing the certificate of fitness to the worker	5
	Explain the fitness advice to the patient: He is able to do so by arranging his workstation in such a way as to avoid jolting and prolonged sitting in a non-ergonomic position (including the seat): by allowing him short rest periods (10 minutes every two hours) during which he can relax and loosen his back muscles. If necessary, he should be assigned to a workstation that avoids heavy loads and whole-body vibrations transmitted by the seat.	10
Patient education		**60**
	Regular, long-term physical exercise and spinal conservation techniques	10
	Resuming physical activity and a socio-professional life without apprehension	5
	Take 15-minute breaks every two hours (when traveling), during which he can relax and loosen his back muscles.	10
	Frequent changes in posture	5
	Avoid prolonged sitting	10
	Show the patient how to handle loads ergonomically	10
	Communicating understandable information to the patient	10

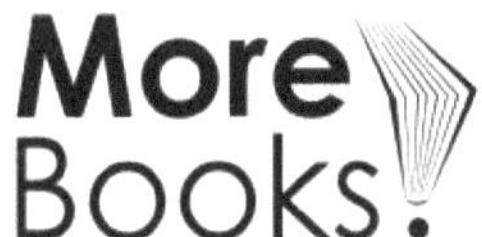

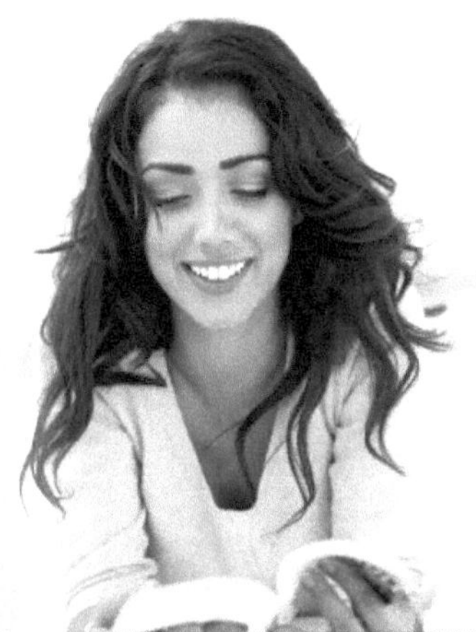

I want morebooks!

Buy your books fast and straightforward online - at one of world's fastest growing online book stores! Environmentally sound due to Print-on-Demand technologies.

Buy your books online at
www.morebooks.shop

Kaufen Sie Ihre Bücher schnell und unkompliziert online – auf einer der am schnellsten wachsenden Buchhandelsplattformen weltweit! Dank Print-On-Demand umwelt- und ressourcenschonend produziert.

Bücher schneller online kaufen
www.morebooks.shop

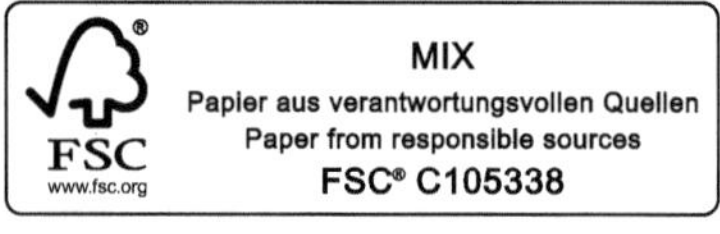

Printed by Books on Demand GmbH, Norderstedt / Germany